# TAKE ME TO THE
# DISPENSARY

Your Quick Guide To Purchasing & Using
Hemp & Cannabis Products

JESSICA FALEIDE, CA

Take Me To The Dispensary
Your Quick Guide To Purchasing & Using Hemp & Cannabis Products
Published in Bottineau, North Dakota USA
www.OrganicWayofLifeLLC.com

Author: Jessica Faleide
Editor: Shelly Sears Moltzen
Formatter: Robin Reed
Front & Back Cover Design: Jessica Faleide, Graphics Plus
Illustration: Tisserand Institute, Jessica Faleide
Publisher: Organic Way of Life, LLC through Self Publishing School

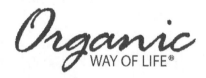

Library of Congress Control Number: 2023903797
Paperback ISBN: 979-8-9878458-0-6
Kindle ISBN: 979-8-9878458-1-3

# Get Your Free Gift!

As a thank you, I've created a one-page quick guide to bring with you to make your trip to the dispensary even easier!

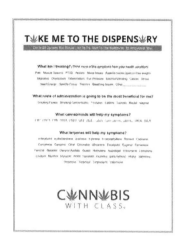

You can download and print a copy by visiting:

# www.TakeMeToTheDispensary.com

# DEDICATION

*This book is dedicated to all of the people who have hope for healing. I don't know you personally or your specific health condition you are currently battling, but know there are people who are here to assist you on your journey as you experience the healing power of hemp and cannabis.*

*I want to thank my parents Erling and Linda Faleide and family friend Leland Hagen for your unending support and encouragement in my healing journey.*

*To all of you reading this, I am so honored to be a part of your healing journey! xoxo*

# IF YOU ARE
# READY TO
# **SPEED UP**
# YOUR HEALING
# **NOW**

Watch 3 Minute Video How It Works:
www.IncreaseBloodFlowAndOxygen.com

Next Watch 8 Minute Video How It's Used:
www.16minutesAday.com

**www.EnhanceLocalBloodFlow.com**

# TABLE OF CONTENTS

# INTRODUCTION

As a medical cannabis patient, clinical aromatherapist and cannabis product formulator, when I've sat in the dispensary waiting rooms and listened to first time medical cannabis patients, so many people were overwhelmed and confused about what they needed, what cannabis was going to do for them and how to take it.

This quick guide was something I felt could be a simple start for all you newbies to help you know what questions you should ask and to be able to effectively communicate with the budtenders what you need and want to achieve with your cannabis or hemp goals.

With the cannabis and hemp industry rising, and with the variety of cannabis products you can purchase, it can be an overwhelming experience stepping into a dispensary, especially for the first time. I want to help you make the best decision on what you want for your specific issue so you can get the most effective results from your selections.

My goal with this quick guide was to break it down to the bare minimum information to make your experience intentional. Even though the budtenders are there to assist you with all of your questions, this can serve them better if you are clear on your intention for being there. The main two questions are: "What are your symptoms that you are trying to relieve?" and "How do you want to take your plant product?"

The following chapters will break down the basics on why you are there, what you want to achieve, what terpenes and cannabinoids will be the most effective, how long do you need the benefits to last and which route of administration will get you there?

Let's get to it!

# BASIC TERMS TO KNOW AT THE DISPENSARY

**CANNABIS-** Contains more than 0.3% THC along with a full range of phytocannabinoids, terpenes, flavonoids, fatty acids and phytochemicals.

**HEMP-** Contains under 0.3% THC along with a full range of phytocannabinoids, terpenes, flavonoids, fatty acids and phytochemicals.

**FULL SPECTRUM-** Contains all the parts of the plant including THC.

**BROAD SPECTRUM-** Contains all the parts of the plant minus THC.

**ISOLATE-** Contains only one cannabinoid. There are no other parts of the plant present. (ex CBD Isolate)

**DISTILLATE-** A thick, golden liquid created by refining cannabis resin. Distillation allows the processor to isolate a desired compound from the cannabis plant and leave behind undesirable plant material. Used inside vape cartridges. They also tend to be potent because they isolate a specific compound that was of high concentration.

**OIL-** A liquid extract used in tinctures, capsules, vaping or for topical preparations.

**TERPENE-** Highly aromatic compounds found in plants and herbs that affect aroma, color and taste. Not to be confused with cannabinoids. Products containing just terpenes are legal in areas where some cannabinoids are not.

**TERPENOIDS-** Any of a class of hydrocarbons that consist of terpenes attached to an oxygen containing group.

**CANNABINOIDS**- Compounds in the cannabis plant (ex. CBD, THC, THCA) which have the ability to interact with cannabinoid receptors in your body's endocannabinoid system.

## CANNABIS CHEMOVARS

TYPE 1- THC Dominant

TYPE 2- Balanced Ratio THC and CBD

TYPE 3- CBD Dominant

*Due to so many cannabis hybrids, industry standards in most states no longer go by Cannabis Sativa and Indica, they go by Chemovar Types 1-3.*

# WHAT IS YOUR PURPOSE?

## *Recreational or Medical*

The first question you need to ask yourself is, "Why am I going to the dispensary?" Are you a recreational cannabis or hemp user or a medical cannabis patient trying to help relieve symptoms from a specific health condition?

**If you are a recreational user, what is your goal?**

Do you care about:

- Taste
- What form the cannabis comes in (dry herb, concentrates, tinctures, edibles)
- How long you do want the effects to last?
- What route of administration do you want to take cannabis/hemp? Do you want to smoke it, apply it topically or ingest it?
- Do you want THC?
- Do you want something that is a one-time use or for the plant material to last a certain amount of time?
- What is legal in your state or region where you live? Cannabis, Hemp, CBD Isolate, or only terpenes?
- What is your budget?

**If you are a medical cannabis patient, these should be the questions you need to ask yourself.**

You should care about:

- Taste
- What type of cannabis product are you willing to try? (dry herb, concentrates, tinctures, edibles)
- How long you do need the effects to last?

- What route of administration do you want to take cannabis? Do you want to smoke it, apply it topically, ingest it or all three?
- Do you need THC?
- Are you dealing with an acute or chronic issue? Meaning, is this a temporary situation or long-term chronic condition you are treating?
- What is legal in your state or region where you live? Are you able to purchase Cannabis (THC content over 0.3%), Hemp (THC under 0.3%) or are you only able to use terpenes?
- What is your budget?
- What is the legal amount of cannabis you can have in possession with your medical card?

# A QUICK BREAKDOWN FOR MEDICAL CANNABIS PATIENTS

## TASTE

Taste is such a controversial topic, and everyone has their own opinion if it should matter or not. This may not seem to be important, but there actually is a reason you should care about the taste. If you don't care for the taste, and if it's for long term use, you are not going to want to take your medical cannabis, therefore, not get benefits. Also, when you dread taking your products, you are making it a negative experience psychologically.

When we are on a healing journey, you should try to make every part of it a positive experience, and like it or not, the flavor of the cannabis you are taking makes a difference psychologically, which makes a difference physically.

If it's short term, most people can suck it up (pun intended), even if they don't like the taste. When you know your cannabis product has all the medicinal compounds in it that are specifically beneficial for your condition, you can usually get through it. When you know the end is short term, it makes it easier to continue, even if it's not enjoyable.

The nice thing if you don't care for the taste, there are options in making it more enjoyable. If you are infusing your own dry herb to make a tincture, I love infusing dry herb into a flavored olive oil such as blood orange and lime. I usually purchase these from wineries that grow their own olive trees.

Another option is purchasing liquid terpenes to adjust taste and therapeutic benefits. There are brands that are made to be taken internally, and some that are not. This is very important to know when researching terpenes.

What I DO NOT recommend is using essential oils to add to your oral products. Unless you are a Clinical Internal Aromatherapist, DO NOT GO THERE!

## WHAT TYPE OF CANNABIS PRODUCTS ARE YOU WILLING TO TRY?

When it all comes down to it, you need to buy something that you will use and use it properly. No matter how much pain you are in, if you bought a suppository that will relieve the pain, but there is no way in hell you are going to stick a little hard cannabis infused cocoa butter object inside your rectum, just looking at it won't relieve your pain. You have to actually use it to get benefits.

Also keep in mind your physical or health limitations. If you have emphysema and can barely breathe, smoking probably shouldn't be your first option. You may want to do a tincture or edible.

If you have physical hand issues, rolling a joint and trying to light it will not be convenient or safe. You don't need to start a house fire in the process of lighting it. Maybe a vape pen, edible or tincture may work best for you.

I also recommend selecting for your symptoms, not your health condition. The reason being is because everyone with the same condition doesn't always experience the same symptoms. For example, having migraines. Not everyone vomits when they have migraines. You may experience them differently than others do.

Another factor is depending on where you live, the selection of cannabis will vary with what products are going to be available to you. Edibles are still illegal currently in some states that have approved cannabis medically legal.

Whatever your health condition and symptoms you experience from it, the form the cannabis comes in does make a difference.

Basically, this goes hand in hand with route of administration, the strength of the cannabis, concentration of cannabinoids, especially THC content, and what you need it to do are all important.

These are all factors that will determine the type of cannabis and product you should purchase.

## HOW LONG DO YOU NEED THE EFFECTS TO LAST?

If you prefer taking your cannabis product fewer times a day, oral products will be better if you stay on top of your dosing. If you want or need inhalation, your effects will be quicker. However, the cannabis compounds will be metabolized and eliminated quicker from your body, therefore you will be inhaling more often during the day to keep the compounds in the therapeutic window. Repeating inhalation more often is necessary to have maximum efficacy in your body.

Remember more is not better, especially when it comes to THC. Sometimes microdosing more often is more effective than taking one big puff of a concentrate once a day. If you are going to bed, and need the effects to last throughout the night to help you sleep and stay asleep, I would time your dosing so that the effects will start to take place once you're in bed sleeping.

For example, you can't sleep due to pain and you want to go to bed at 9pm. If you had an edible that was for pain and contained THC, and you didn't want to experience the feeling of being high, I would take that edible 1 ½ to 2 hours before bed. In this example that would be 7-7:30pm when you would eat your edible, then lay down for bed at 9pm.

This way the effects will start to kick in, but the psychoactive effects won't be felt because you will be sleeping. The full duration of the effects will be helping to minimize your pain during the 5-8 hours while you are asleep. When you awake, you can take another form of cannabis during the day.

# WHAT ROUTE OF ADMINISTRATION DO YOU WANT TO TAKE YOUR HEMP OR CANNABIS?

Do you want to smoke it, apply it topically, administer under your tongue or swallow it? Do you need multiple routes at once throughout the day? Depending on your health condition, I recommend multiple cannabis products in different forms and routes of administration.

For example, if you have physical pain, and say you also experience random muscle spasms and need immediate relief, I would use a cannabis product I could smoke for immediate relief, but also have a topical on the areas of pain, along with microdosing with a tincture throughout the day to stay ahead of the pain.

These all have different absorption and duration times. This is why I would take that approach. When one wears off, the other has kicked in. The best protocol is to stay ahead of the pain, but have a backup for immediate relief, hence smoking. Whether you prefer a vape pen which is more concentrated or dry herb to smoke in a joint or pipe, this is a nice backup plan for those emergency moments.

# DO YOU NEED THC?

*Hemp below 0.3% THC or Cannabis above 0.3% THC*

Again, this depends where you live and if you even need THC for your symptoms. If you do need THC, you must be aware of how your body responds to THC and make sure you start low and go slow. Start with lower THC concentration and dose fewer times a day starting out. More is not better!

Everyone's endocannabinoid system is different and responds different to cannabis, especially THC. It's amazing how a little THC can be beneficial, but even at a low dose you can still get high easily. If you don't do well with the psychoactive effects, you need to learn how to properly take THC and know your limits.

The main effect of THC is what is commonly referred to as "couch lock." We want to help minimize the feeling of immobility. There are ways to counteract couch lock, short term memory loss, paranoia and the feeling of being high while still taking THC and still be a functioning human being.

One recommendation to decrease the feeling of being high or paranoia is by taking a CBD isolate tincture to counteract the effects of THC. This is not to be confused with hemp extract. (Hemp extract will potentially enhance your high depending on the CBD mg. I have found a hemp extract that contains over 66mg CBD per 1mL, and it was effective for me personally in cutting the high.)

For flower, having a nice 50/50 blend of THC and CBD will help lower the longevity of being high.

Another tip to reduce the psychoactive effects of THC is to use products that contain terpenes such as myrcene, linalool, limonene or a-pinene to help minimize the sensations and shorten the longevity of being high.

When THC and myrcene synergistically work together, they create a sedation effect which minimizes the feeling of immobility.

Alpha pinene will help to shorten the effect of memory loss from THC. Linalool is a strong an antianxiety agent without producing a lot of sedation on its own and counteracts the anxiogenic tendencies like paranoia caused by THC. As far as limonene, it is currently being researched and showing promising results to help reduce anxiety and paranoia.

## ARE YOU DEALING WITH AN ACUTE OR CHRONIC ISSUE?

To simplify this question, are you dealing with a temporary condition or situation or a long-term chronic condition?

The amount of plant material you purchase can corollate with the length of time you will be using cannabis. If you broke a bone and are taking cannabis for pain, this is a short term condition. Your pain with bone healing will only be a few weeks.

If you have cancer, this will be something you are treating for a longer period of time with multiple issues like, nausea, vomiting and possibly need the cannabis strain to stimulate appetite.

If this is long term, find a product you feel comfortable in getting into a routine using. If you are a recovering alcoholic or currently struggling with alcohol use, I wouldn't purchase a tincture that was alcohol based. I would stick to an oil-based tincture such as olive oil or MCT oil. If you can't purchase an oil based tincture, I suggest making your own. If you live in a state where you can legally make your own, that is probably the best option. This way you can control what is in your tincture.

## WHAT IS LEGAL IN YOUR STATE OR REGION WHERE YOU LIVE?

Are you able to purchase cannabis (THC content over 0.3%), hemp (THC under 0.3%) or are you only able to use terpenes? If you have a medical cannabis card, this allows you to legally purchase THC products when you aren't in a recreational state.

Due to the current laws, in some places even CBD isolate is illegal. Just because you live in an area where cannabis and hemp are legal, where you work and if you are drug tested can play a big role in your options for cannabis.

Even though hemp products should contain below 0.3% THC, that doesn't mean the lab testing it had used up to date testing equipment. That product you purchased could actually contain a higher percentage than what was shown on the product label. Therefore, your job position could be in danger if your blood test said you were above the legal limits of THC in your system.

## WHAT IS YOUR BUDGET?

Let's be honest, medical bills add up, and when you have to pay out of pocket to purchase cannabis for medicine, it can get expensive! What you are financially able to spend will play a big part in what you are going to purchase.

If you are smoking, and on a budget, herb is lower in price along with vape pen cartridges. However, with herb, what you are smoking it out of can vary big time from papers, pipes, bongs, to electric apparatuses that can be more than you budgeted for. Then we have concentrates which tend to have a higher price point along with what you use to vape them from.

However, it can be cheaper in the long run if you are going to be using these apparatuses for a longer period of time. I also like electric apparatuses if you are using herb and concentrates, because the temperatures are preset to give you the best benefits from your plant material.

This means you will need less product because you aren't burning the compounds with too high of heat, getting less benefit. When you burn at the right temperature, you need less cannabis and the effects are more potent. Therefore, you won't have to buy more product as frequently. This means better effect, less product= save money.

## WHAT IS THE LEGAL AMOUNT OF CANNABIS YOU ARE ALLOWED IN YOUR POSSESSION?

Depending on your health condition, that may determine the amount of cannabis you are able to purchase in a month with your medical card (If you are in a medical only area). This means you are allotted so many ounces/grams a month per patient.

People with chronic health conditions such as cancer usually are able to purchase a larger volume of cannabis products with their card due to the fact they may need more cannabis, more frequently to relieve their symptoms.

# CANNABIS PRODUCTS

**Inhalation (Smokeable):**

Dry Herb:
    Trim/Shake
    Bud/Flower
    Kief

Concentrates: (but not limited to)
    Resin/Wax
    Diamonds
    Budder/Badder
    Distillates/Oil
    Shatter/Shadder
    Isolates
    Flan™

**Oral:**

Edibles (gummies, brownies, cookies, candy)
Tinctures (can be oil or alcohol based)
Liquid Beverages
Capsules
RSO

**Buccal/Sublingual:**

Tinctures
Pouches

**Topical:**

Transdermal patches
Lotion
Balms
Gels

Sprays
Massage Oils
RSO

**Rectal:**

Suppositories

**Vaginal:**

Pessaries

# ROUTES OF ADMINISTRATION

The amount of time cannabis can take effect is going to be a little different for each individual. Everyone's endocannabinoid system is different, so everyone will respond differently. The times given in the next pages ahead regarding effects and duration are going to be on average what people may experience.

Also, what you have eaten and how quickly your body metabolizes compounds in the liver will make a difference on the duration of effects. If you take cannabis after eating a fatty meal or snacks, the effects will last longer because it will be in your system longer. The compounds are going to continue circulating in the body until they are metabolized into water soluble metabolites to be eliminated via feces or urine.

If you are a recreational user and used to high concentrations of THC and take cannabis frequently throughout the day, the amount of time it takes effect will be different from a new person just trying cannabis for the first time for medical issues because of your endocannabinoid system.

For topical application, the effects can also vary depending on skin ethnicity, your genetic sex, type of skin (dry, oily, compromised), if the skin is warm, location of topical product on the body, and if the product is occluded. Another determination is what other compounds are in your topical product. Some terpenes can help enhance penetration into the skin. There are many factors that determine the dosage to stay in the therapeutic window of efficacy. Another factor is how many times you are applying the topical or if it is a transdermal patch where it can stay on the skin for around 12 hours and is time released.

When using suppositories (rectal) or pessaries (vaginal) there are also factors to take into consideration of how long they will take effect. What is the base ingredient, are you laying down and going to bed, or are you walking around with it in during the day? What is the concentration of cannabis or terpenes in the product? These are all factors along with your endocannabinoid system and if you are new to cannabis on the duration of effects with both of these products.

## THERAPEUTIC WINDOW

Therapeutic Window For Dosing and Half-Life

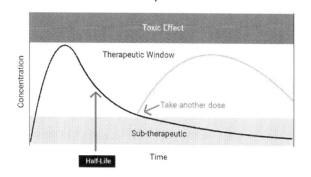

*(Graph by Tisserand Institute)*

What in the world do I mean when I am talking about therapeutic window? This means the dose range of a drug (or plant-based product) that provides safe and effective therapy with minimal adverse effects.

When I talk about therapeutic window for dosing, the picture above can give you a visual of what that means. When looking at the routes of administration and the amount of time it takes to feel the effects and the duration of how long the effects are going to last, this is the reason why we need to keep dosing. The goal is to keep the cannabis compounds into the bloodstream for maximum efficacy.

What is half-life? It's the time it takes for the amount of an orally taken drug's active substance in your body to reduce by half. Half-life takes place once the compounds go through the liver and are metabolized. Each time the blood circulates, the compounds are going to be half as effective each pass through the liver until that metabolite is able to be eliminated from the body.

The fascinating thing is, taking THC orally has a different effect. Most compound's effects are minimized after metabolism, but the metabolite of THC is actually more potent after it's metabolized in the liver. This is why oral ingestion is more potent than smoking. With smoking, you don't have first pass metabolism as you do with oral ingestion. When you smoke, the compounds are directly absorbed into your bloodstream before it passes through your liver.

Let's walk through an example of smoking to keep you into the therapeutic window of efficacy. Say you smoked a joint and it took 5 minutes to take effect. Then say one hour later was the peak of the pain relief and highest you got. After 2 hours you are feeling even less, and in another hour, you really aren't feeling the effects.

Before you get to where the effects have worn off, this is when you want to take another puff. You want take another puff before you get out of the sub-therapeutic window and where you are no longer feeling any therapeutic effects. This would mean you need to take another puff 3 hours after your first inhalation in this example to stay in the therapeutic window. Does this make sense? Feel free to revisit these pages to visually understand dosing.

Here is another example with oral medicine. Have you ever had surgery and were prescribed pain pills? Let's say you were prescribed to take one pill every 3 hours to relieve your pain. Then you went to bed for 9 hours and woke up in extreme pain. This is why. It's because you had been consistent in taking the prescription every 3 hours to keep the prescription in your blood stream in the therapeutic window.

When you went to bed, you weren't dosing because you were sleeping and then the prescription fell below the sub-therapeutic window to being completely eliminated from your body due to continued half-life. Now you aren't feeling any benefits from the prescription. It's like taking a photo copy of a photo copy, and a copy of the last copy and so on until you can't even see the font from the original sheet.

It is important that you must keep dosing and in the right time frame to keep the cannabis working at full efficacy for your symptoms. Each route will have different amounts of time to stay in the therapeutic window and you will see this for each route in the next chapters.

It's also wise to keep a journal since every body is different in how quickly we metabolize cannabinoids, terpenes and other compounds.

# INHALATION/ SMOKING

**How long to take effect:**
Immediately to 15 minutes

**Duration of effect:**
2-4 hours

**Ways to smoke:**
Preroll/Joint, Pipe, Bong, One-hitter, Vaporizer, Vape Pen

**How to use:**

Whether you are inhaling dry herb or concentrates, always start low and go slow. Start with herb before concentrates when smoking cannabis. It's recommended to start with one puff before inhaling a second. With herb inhale through your mouth, and exhale through your mouth. Wait 5 minutes to see how your body is responding before you take that second inhale. This is not like a cigarette. You do not need to hold in the smoke in your mouth and lungs to get benefits. When inhaling terpenes, we know absorption through the oral mucosa is very good. The dose with inhalation will depend on how deep and for how long you inhale the smoke or vapors.

When using a vape pen, you will take this in a different way. As for vape oil, there is a technique to make your inhalation more effective. You're going to inhale through your mouth then exhale through your nose. This way you are getting absorption in your mouth (oral mucosa), through your lungs, you're psychologically benefiting from the aroma in your nasal passage, and then you swallow the compounds. This technique will increase the efficacy of the vape oil preparation.

Journal how long it took to feel the effects, how long it lasted, what you ate prior and what product you used to find what works the best for you. It may take testing multiple strains to find the best product for you and your symptoms if you are smoking for medicinal purposes.

# ORAL

**How long to take effect:**
30-180 minutes

**Duration of effect:**
5-8 hours

**Product Types:**
Edibles, Liquid Beverages, Capsules, RSO (Rick Simpson Oil)

**How to use:**

Liquid beverages currently are basically CBD. They are not formulated to help heal a health condition. Check the label for ingredients.

The potency of edibles will vary if you make your own or purchase from the dispensary. Start low and go slow. Especially if you are ingesting THC. Due to the length of time it takes for it to reach your liver to be metabolized, some people think it isn't doing anything and eat more. Do not do this. When you eat an edible, THC is converted into a stronger metabolite called 11-Hydroxy-THC making you even higher than if you smoked cannabis with THC. Journal what you ate and how much you consumed if eating an edible with THC.

Even though RSO is called an oil, it is a thick distillate. You can use RSO to make an edible, take it with food or dilute with MCT or olive oil to make a tincture. However, there is an easier way to dose and take this orally. Take a piece of wax paper and syringe the RSO in a line on the wax paper. Place in the freezer until it's hard. Take a knife and cut the now hardened distillate into pieces the thickness of a toothpick. This is highly concentrated THC, so start with one sliver of RSO at a time. Put the distillate back in the freezer in an airtight container or ziplock bag. Get instructions on dosing from your cannabis doctor.

# TAKE ME TO THE DISPENSARY

*Do not inhale RSO due to the high concentration of THC, the presence of other plant compounds that should not be inhaled, along with residual solvent from the cannabinoid extraction process.*

# BUCCAL/SUBLINGUAL
Between your cheek and gumline / under the tongue

**How long to take effect:**
15-20 minutes

**Duration of effect:**
4-6 hours

**Product types:**
Tinctures, Hard candy to suck on, Pouches

**How to use:**

Tinctures are taken by using the calibrated dropper measured with the appropriate dose of liquid, then drop that amount of product under your tongue or in between your lower gum line and cheeks. Hold the drops in your mouth for 30 seconds to a minute to allow the compounds to absorb into your bloodstream before you swallow your saliva.

Oil based tinctures are better for absorption of terpenes and cannabinoids because they are administered in the presence of fat (oil) which increases the absorption and is more preferable. This is also better on your oral mucosa. With alcohol-based tinctures, the repeat dosing (under your tongue or gumline) on your mucosa can be harmful.

You can put the hard candy between your gums and cheek also, or suck on it until it dissolves and penetrates into your bloodstream. When you swallow your saliva, the residual compounds will also be ingested.

Put the pouch between your cheek and gums. Follow manufacturer's guideline for length of time. I wouldn't recommend placing the pouches in the exact same place in your cheek every time. Insert the pouches to different areas of your cheeks and sides to give your mucosa a break.

# TOPICAL

**How long to take effect:**
Transdermal patches 30-45 minutes
Liquids, Gels, Lotion: Varies
Creams, Oils, Balms: Varies
RSO: Varies

**Duration of effect:**
Transdermal patches: 5-12 hours
Liquids, Gels, Lotion: Varies
Creams, Oils, Balms: Varies
RSO: Varies

**Product Types:**
Sprays, Gels, Lotion, Cream, Oil, Balm, Transdermal Patches, RSO (Rick Simpson Oil)

**How to use:**

Transdermal patch- Apply to clean, dry, hairless skin, without cuts, rashes or cracked. Apply in an area with good circulation and where it won't rub off. You can apply to your lower back, inner thigh, abdomen, or wrist. Always follow manufacturer's guideline for application and duration time. These are not your best option due to how they release into the body. You tend to get minimal results with cannabinoids and terpenes in this form delivered through a patch. Hydrogels and lotions are more effective with cannabis and terpene delivery.

If you are allergic or sensitive to adhesives, transdermal patches may not be the best option. If you apply a patch and you start to itch and get a rash or hives, remove the patch and wash your skin with soap and water immediately.

If you do use a patch, try it by itself first to see how you respond before incorporating a tincture or edible in the mix right away. Once you know how you respond to multiple methods separately, then you can dose with multiple products when you monitor each route's therapeutic window of efficacy.

As far as topicals from sprays, gels, lotion, balms or oils, the duration is going to depend on the base, the cannabinoids and the terpene blend in the formula. The synergy of the components in the formula makes a huge difference in the efficacy of what you are treating.

Also the base of what the terpenes and cannabinoids are in effect penetration. Spray, gels and lotions penetrate quicker, whereas thicker creams and oils take longer to penetrate. You must keep reapplying throughout the day to keep the compounds in your system in the therapeutic window to be effective.

To use RSO topically, syringe a small amount of RSO onto the area that is being treated. Place a bandage (occlusion) over the area. If you are using the RSO *neat* (undiluted) and if your skin feels irritated, you can dilute the RSO with hemp seed oil (not hemp extract), olive oil, MCT or fractionated coconut oil. Repeat topical application as directed from your cannabis doctor.

# RECTAL

**How long to take effect:**
5 minutes and up

**Duration of effect:**
Varies

**Product Types:**
Suppositories

**How to use:**

Insert suppository up inside your rectum at least fingernail depth. It is best to insert when you know you will be laying down for an extended period of time, bedtime is ideal.

It's good to have a panty liner or underwear protector so the ingredients don't stain your sheets, clothes or underwear. Most suppositories are cocoa butter based and melt when in contact with warm temperature; therefore, it doesn't take long for the suppository to melt and the compounds start to absorb. The rectum has 2 routes of absorption.

Journal the time you inserted it to when you started to feel benefits, and when the benefits started to wear off. Obviously, if you are sleeping you may not know the timeline of efficacy and when it wore off.

# VAGINAL

**How long to take effect:**
5 minutes and up

**Duration of effect:**
Varies

**Product Types:**
Pessary

**How to use:**

Insert pessary into the vagina. Insert to the depth of where the bottom of an inserted tampon would end. It is best to insert a pessary at night or when you're going to be laying down for a longer period of time. This is so the product doesn't melt and run out of your body before the compounds are able to be absorbed into your bloodstream. It is recommended to wear a panty liner or to protect your undergarments to prevent staining from certain ingredients like cocoa butter.

Journal the time you inserted it to when you started to feel benefits, and when the benefits started to wear off. Obviously, if you are sleeping you may not know the timeline of efficacy and when it wore off.

# CANNABINOIDS

## Therapeutic Benefits Of Each Cannabinoid

### CBC *Cannabichromene*

- Pain relief
- Slows bacterial growth
- Reduces swelling/inflammation
- Inhibits cancer cell growth
- Promotes bone growth
- Inhibits growth of fungus

### CBCA *Cannabichromenic Acid*

- Pain relief
- Reduces swelling/inflammation
- Active against acne bacteria
- Reduces symptoms of depression
- Positive impact on brain cells

# CBD *Cannabidiol*

- Reduces the feeling of being high from THC
- Pain relief when formulated with other compounds (terpenes or cannabinoids)
- Slows bacterial growth
- Reduces blood sugar issues
- Reduces symptoms of depression
- Reduces nausea and vomiting
- Reduces seizures & convulsions
- Reduces swelling/inflammation
- Improves sleep
- Inhibits cancer cell growth
- Calming
- Prevents muscle spasms
- Reduces symptoms of anxiety
- Promotes bone growth
- Reduces intestinal spasms associated with IBS
- Slows nervous system deterioration
- Active against p. acnes bacteria

# CBDA *Cannabidiolic acid*

- Slows bacterial growth
- Reduces seizures & convulsions

# CBDV *Cannabidivarin*

- Promotes bone growth
- Decreases appetite

## CBG *Cannabigerol*

- Slows bacterial growth
- Reduces swelling/inflammation
- Inhibits cancer cell growth
- Promotes bone growth

## CBGA *Cannabigerolic acid*

- Slows bacterial growth
- Reduces swelling/inflammation
- Inhibits cancer cell growth

## CBGV *Cannabigerovarin*

- Pain relief
- Reduces swelling/inflammation
- Prevents muscle spasms

# CBN *Cannabinol*

* Pain relief
* Improves sleep (only when combined with certain terpenes)
* Prevents muscle spasms

## **D8 THC** *Delta-8 Tetrahydrocannabinol*

- Provides less of a high than delta-9 THC
- Protects nerve cells against damage, degeneration or impairment function
- Increases appetite
- Reduce nausea and vomiting
- Reduces symptoms of anxiety
- Pain relief
- Reduces swelling/inflammation

*"But there are potential safety concerns. As with Delta-9, Russo says, Delta-8 can cause issues such as toxic psychosis when consumed in large amounts. Poor quality control and fake product labels are other issues that can come up in the marketplace."*

*– Dr. Ethan Russo, M.D.*

## **D9 THC** *Delta-9 Tetrahydrocannabinol*

- Will get you high and can cause couch lock, short term memory loss, and paranoia
- Pain relief
- Reduces symptoms of depression
- Reduces nausea and vomiting
- Increases appetite
- Prevents muscle spasms
- Reduces stress
- Reduces eye pressure
- Reduces swelling/inflammation

# THCA *Tetrahydrocannabinolic Acid*

- Reduces swelling/inflammation
- Inhibits cancer cell growth
- Prevents muscle spasms
- Protects nerve cells against damage, degeneration or impairment function
- Reduces nausea & vomiting

# THCV *Tetrahydrocannabivarin*

- Enhances effect of THC, but minimizes the longevity of the high
- Reduces blood sugar issues
- Reduces seizures & convulsions
- Improves focus
- Increases energy
- Promotes bone growth
- Appetite suppressant

# THC-O *THC acetate ester*

- No benefits. Stick with delta-9 THC.

*"So, between the inherent danger of the process to make it, the potential toxicity of the product, and its illegality, I've got to recommend that people forget about it. It's just not something that people should be trying." - Dr. Ethan Russo, M.D.*

# TERPENES/TERPENOIDS

## Alpha bisabolol (a-bisabolol)

Smell/Taste: Earthy, Floral, Herbal, Peppery

Therapeutic Benefits

* Reduces swelling/inflammation
* Reduces symptoms of anxiety
* Pain relief
* Protects nerve cells against damage, degeneration or impairment function
* Inhibits growth of fungus
* Stops or kills microorganisms from growing and causing disease
* Free radical scavenging activity
* Reduces and stops infections by parasites
* Relieves itching
* Relieves spasms from voluntary or involuntary muscles
* Stops abnormal cell growth
* Prevents the onset of ulcers
* Cell regenerative for skin, scar and wound healing
* Skin penetration enhancer
* Inhibits cancer cells in the brain and spinal cord
* Reduces gastric lesions. Can be used in the treatment of alcoholism.
* Promotor of programmed cell death for human leukemia cells
* Blocks the sensation of pain to your brain, providing you pain relief

# Alpha phellandrene (a-phellandrene)

Smell/Taste: Earthy, Floral, Fruity, Herbal

<u>Therapeutic Benefits</u>

- Reduces swelling/inflammation
- Destructive to bacteria
- Reduces symptoms of depression
- Stops heightened sensitivity to pain
- Blocks the sensation of pain to your brain, providing you pain relief
- Relieves spasms from voluntary or involuntary muscles
- Stops abnormal cell growth
- Stimulates functioning of the immune system
- Free radical scavenging activity
- Inhibits growth of fungus

# Alpha pinene (a-pinene)

Smell/Taste: Pine, Balsam, Woody, Turpentine

Therapeutic Benefits

- Pain relief
- Destructive to bacteria
- Inhibits growth of fungus (candida)
- Reduces swelling/inflammation
- Blocks the sensation of pain to your brain, providing you pain relief
- Relieves spasms from voluntary or involuntary muscles
- Inhibits growth of viruses
- Reduces symptoms of anxiety
- Counteracts gastric mucosal damage
- Prevents bone loss
- Inhibits cancer cells
- Free radical scavenging activity
- Decreases heart rate from stress
- Shortens the effect of memory loss from THC

# Beta pinene (b-pinene)

Smell/Taste: Citrus, Earthy, Floral

Therapeutic Benefits

- Reduces swelling/inflammation
- Destructive to bacteria
- Inhibits growth of fungus (candida)
- Blocks the sensation of pain to your brain, providing you pain relief
- Free radical scavenging activity
- Relieves spasms from voluntary or involuntary muscles
- Prevents bone loss

# Beta-caryophyllene (b-caryophyllene)

Smell/Taste: Earthy, Floral, Fruity

Therapeutic Benefits

* Pain relief
* Reduces swelling/inflammation
* Destructive to bacteria
* Acts against biofilms (plaque forming bacteria like on teeth)
* Blocks the sensation of pain to your brain, providing you pain relief
* Relieves spasms from voluntary or involuntary muscles
* Stops abnormal cell growth
* Inhibits growth of viruses
* Reduces the symptoms of anxiety
* Helps your immune system self regulate to adjust to immune responses
* Local anesthesia
* Protects nerve cells against damage, degeneration or impairment function
* Protection against heart disease and atherosclerosis
* Inhibits cancer cell growth
* Used to safely wean addicts from drugs and alcohol

# Borneol

Smell/Taste: Mint, Camphor, Menthol

<u>Therapeutic Benefits</u>

- Reduces swelling/inflammation
- Destructive to bacteria
- Inhibits the coagulation of blood
- Inhibits growth of fungus
- Free radical scavenging activity
- Relieves spasms from voluntary or involuntary muscles
- Inhibits growth of viruses
- Cell regenerative for skin, scar and wound healing
- Stops excitation of a nerve after transmission of an impulse
- Protects nerve cells against damage, degeneration or impairment function
- Prevents bone loss
- Calming
- Pain relief

# Cadinene

Smell/Taste: Citrus, Earthy, Floral, Herbal

Therapeutic Benefits

- Destructive to bacteria
- Stops abnormal cell growth
- Reduces swelling/inflammation
- Free radical scavenging activity

# Camphene

Smell/Taste: Citrus, Floral, Herbal

<u>Therapeutic Benefits</u>

- Reduces swelling/inflammation
- Blocks the sensation of pain to your brain, providing you pain relief
- Free radical scavenging activity
- Breaks down mucus
- Destructive to bacteria
- Lowers cholesterol
- Repairs bone
- Used in treatment for Alzheimer's
- Used for liver cell damage

# Camphor

Smell/Taste: Woody, Mint

<u>Therapeutic Benefits</u>

- Pain relief
- Destructive to bacteria
- Inhibits growth of fungus
- Prevents or relieves a cough
- Central nervous system stimulant
- Breaks down mucus
- Prevents bone loss
- Improves blood flow
- Appetite suppressant
- Reduces seizures & convulsions

# Citral

Smell/Taste: Citrus, Floral, Herbal

<u>Therapeutic Benefits</u>

- ♯ Stops or kills airborne microorganisms from growing and causing disease
- ♯ Pain relief
- ♯ Stops pain due to a stimulus that does not normally provoke pain
- ♯ Reduces swelling caused by too much fluid trapped in the body's tissue
- ♯ Reduces swelling/inflammation
- ♯ Destructive to bacteria
- ♯ Reduces seizures & convulsions
- ♯ Inhibits growth of fungus
- ♯ Inhibits growth of fungus (candida)
- ♯ Relieves spasms from voluntary or involuntary muscles
- ♯ Stops abnormal cell growth
- ♯ Inhibits growth of viruses
- ♯ Relieves itching
- ♯ Calming

# Citronellol

Smell/Taste: Citrus, Floral, Herbal

Therapeutic Benefits

- Pain relief
- Reduces swelling/inflammation
- Reduces symptoms of anxiety
- Reduces seizures & convulsions
- Inhibits growth of fungus
- Inhibits growth of fungus (candida)
- Free radical scavenging activity
- Relieves spasms from voluntary or involuntary muscles
- Appetite suppressor
- Central Nervous System depressant
- Lowers blood pressure
- Muscle relaxant

# Delta 3 carene

Smell/Taste: Herbal, Spicy, Woody

<u>Therapeutic Benefits</u>

- Reduces swelling/inflammation
- Stops excitation of a nerve after transmission of an impulse
- Breaks down mucus
- Prevents bone loss
- Memory retention
- Free radical scavenging activity
- Inhibits growth of fungus
- Reduces and stops infections by parasites
- Removes excess fluid (causes dry mouth & eyes)

# Eucalyptol/1,8-Cineole

Smell/Taste: Citrus, Earthy, Herbal

Therapeutic Benefits

- Stops or kills airborne microorganisms from growing and causing disease
- Pain relief
- Reduces swelling/inflammation
- Destructive to bacteria
- Blocks the sensation of pain to your brain, providing you pain relief
- Free radical scavenging activity
- Relieves spasms from voluntary or involuntary muscles
- Inhibits growth of viruses
- Memory retention
- Releases or involves dopamine as a neurotransmitter. Used for treating Parkinson's and certain endocrine disorders.
- Counteracts gastric mucosal damage
- Lowers blood pressure
- Increase cerebral blood flow
- Stops excitation of a nerve after transmission of an impulse
- Breaks down mucus
- Skin penetration enhancer
- Used in the treatment of cancer
- Inhibits the growth of fungus

# Eugenol

Smell/Taste: Earthy, Floral, Herbal

<u>Therapeutic Benefits</u>

- Pain relief
- Potential use for diabetics. It lowers glucose in the blood.
- Reduces swelling/inflammation
- Destructive to bacteria
- Inhibits the coagulation of blood
- Reduces seizures & convulsions
- Inhibits growth of fungus (candida)
- Inhibits the physiological effects of histamine. Used in treating allergies.
- Free radical scavenging activity
- Relieves spasms from voluntary or involuntary muscles
- Prevents clots from forming and growing.
- Stops abnormal cell growth
- Prevents the onset of ulcers
- Inhibits growth of viruses
- Lowers blood pressure
- Liver protective
- Protects nerve cells against damage, degeneration or impairment function
- Helps to dilate blood vessels

# Farnesene

Smell/Taste: Floral, Woody

<u>Therapeutic Benefits</u>

- ❧ Inhibits cancer cell growth
- ❧ Protects nerve cells against damage, degeneration or impairment function

# Fenchol

Smell/Taste: Camphor, Citrus, Woody

<u>Therapeutic Benefits</u>

- ❧ Inhibits growth of fungus
- ❧ Stops or kills microorganisms from growing and causing disease

# Geraniol

Smell/Taste: Citrus, Fruity, Herbal

<u>Therapeutic Benefits</u>

- Stops or kills airborne microorganisms from growing and causing disease
- Destructive to bacteria
- Antibiotic resistance modification
- Inhibits growth of fungus
- Inhibits growth of fungus (candida)
- Free radical scavenging activity
- Relieves spasms from voluntary or involuntary muscles
- Stops abnormal cell growth
- Cooling
- Protects nerve cells against damage, degeneration or impairment function
- Potential use for pancreatic, oral (tongue), liver, renal (kidney), skin and prostate cancer

# Geranyl acetate

Smell/Taste: Floral, Fruity, Lavender

Therapeutic Benefits

* Pain Relief
* Stops or kills microorganisms from growing and causing disease
* Inhibits the growth of fungus (candida)
* Blocks the sensation of pain to your brain, providing you pain relief
* Promotes bile secretion by the liver

# Guaiol

Smell/Taste: Pine

Therapeutic Benefits

* Destructive to bacteria

# Humulene

Smell/Taste: Hops, Spicy, Woody

<u>Therapeutic Benefits</u>

- Reduces swelling/inflammation
- Appetite suppressant
- Pain relief
- Inhibits the growth of fungus (candida)
- Stops abnormal cell growth
- Destructive to bacteria
- Inhibits cancer cell growth
- Potential use for prostate cancer

# Isopulegol

Taste/Smell: Herbal, Mint

<u>Therapeutic Therapy</u>

- Pain relief
- Inhibits growth of fungus
- Reduces seizures & convulsions
- Reduces symptoms of depression

# Limonene (d-limonene)

Smell/Taste: Citrus, Fruity, Herbal

Therapeutic Benefits

- Activates white blood cells
- Pain relief
- Reduces swelling/inflammation
- Destructive to bacteria
- Lowers blood pressure
- Blocks the sensation of pain to your brain, providing you pain relief
- Used to treat obesity (being overweight)
- Free radical scavenging activity
- Stops abnormal cell growth
- Prevents the onset of ulcers
- Reduces the symptoms of anxiety
- A natural cleaning out process of your cells so they can prevent and fight disease
- Helpful effects on the liver
- Stimulates functioning of the immune system
- Skin penetration enhancer
- Reduces eye pressure
- Potential to counteract paranoia from THC

# Limonene (l-limonene)

Smell/Taste: Herbal, Mint, Turpentine

<u>Therapeutic Benefits</u>

- Lowers blood pressure
- Free radical scavenging activity
- Skin penetration enhancer
- Promotes wound healing

# Linalool

Smell/Taste: Citrus, Fruity, Herbal

Therapeutic Benefits

- Stops or kills airborne microorganisms from growing and causing disease
- Pain relief
- Reduces swelling/inflammation
- Reduces symptoms of anxiety
- Destructive to bacteria
- Reduces seizures & convulsions
- Inhibits growth of fungus (candida)
- Blocks the sensation of pain to your brain, providing you pain relief
- Free radical scavenging activity
- Relieves spasms from voluntary or involuntary muscles
- Stops abnormal cell growth
- Inhibits growth of viruses
- Improves memory retention
- Lowers blood pressure
- Stimulates functioning of the immune system
- Calming
- Protects nerve cells against damage, degeneration or impairment function
- Used for carpal tunnel syndrome
- Used in treating liver, lung, and colon cancer
- Topical local pain reliver
- Counteracts paranoia from THC

# Menthol

Smell/Taste: Mint

Therapeutic Benefits

* Pain relief
* Reduces swelling/inflammation
* Destructive to bacteria
* Inhibits the coagulation of blood
* Free radical scavenging activity
* Relieves itching
* Relieves spasms from voluntary or involuntary muscles
* Stops abnormal cell growth
* Prevents or relieves a cough
* Promotes bile secretion by the liver
* Central Nervous System stimulant
* Cooling
* Releases or involves dopamine as a neurotransmitter. Used for treating Parkinson's and certain endocrine disorders.
* Lowers blood pressure
* Skin penetration enhancer
* Inhibits cell growth in prostate cancer

# Myrcene

Smell/Taste: Citrus, Diesel, Fruity, Herbal

Therapeutic Benefits

- Counteracts "couch lock" and paranoia from THC
- Pain relief
- Free radical scavenging activity
- Reduces swelling/inflammation
- Blocks the sensation of pain to your brain, providing you pain relief
- Calming
- Prevents ulcers, especially of the wall of the stomach or duodenum (beginning of small intestine)
- Stops or kills microorganisms from growing and causing disease
- Potential to inhibit breast cancer
- Reduces the effects of organic tissue damage in brain tissue

# Nerol

Smell/Taste: Citrus, Earthy, Fruity, Herbal

Therapeutic Benefits

- Destructive to bacteria
- Inhibits growth of fungus

# Nerolidol

Smell/Taste: Citrus, Diesel, Herbal

Therapeutic Benefits

- Reduces swelling/inflammation
- Destructive to bacteria
- Inhibits growth of fungus
- Reduces and stops infections by parasites
- Relieves spasms from voluntary or involuntary muscles
- Stops abnormal cell growth
- Prevents the onset of ulcers
- Reduces the symptoms of anxiety
- Protects nerve cells against damage, degeneration or impairment function
- Skin penetration enhancer
- Calming

# Ocimene

Smell/Taste: Citrus, Floral, Fruity, Herbal

Therapeutic Benefits

- Inhibits growth of fungus
- Stops abnormal cell growth
- Reduces seizures & convulsions
- Inhibits growth of viruses
- Destructive to bacteria
- Reduces swelling/inflammation
- Inhibits the effects against the cause of sleeping sickness
- Potential use for the treatment of oral, liver, leukemic, melanoma, lung, and colon cancer.

# Para-cymene

Smell/Taste: Citrus, Diesel, Herbal

<u>Therapeutic Benefits</u>

- Pain relief
- Reduces swelling/inflammation
- Destructive to bacteria
- Blocks the sensation of pain to your brain, providing you pain relief
- Inhibits growth of viruses
- Reduces eye pressure
- Stops or kills microorganisms from growing and causing disease
- Inhibits cancer pain (in mice)
- Potential use for treatment of breast, ovarian, brain, lung, colon cancer

# Phytol

Smell/Taste: Floral, Herbal

<u>Therapeutic Benefits</u>

- Reduces swelling/inflammation
- Pain relief
- Free radical scavenging activity
- Reduces the need to scratch from allergies
- Enhances immune system response
- Stops abnormal cell growth
- Reduces selzures & convulsions
- Potential use for the treatment of stomach cancer

# Sabinene

Smell/Taste: Citrus, Herbal, Peppery, Spicy

<u>Therapeutic Benefits</u>

- Reduces swelling/inflammation
- Inhibits growth of fungus
- Free radical scavenging activity
- Stops or kills microorganisms from growing and causing disease
- Destructive to bacteria and for salmonella infections
- Calming
- Prevents the reduction of muscle mass
- Inhibits cell growth in colon cancer cells

# Terpinene

Taste/Smell: Citrus, Spicy, Turpentine, Woody

Therapeutic Benefits

- Reduces swelling/inflammation
- Free radical scavenging activity
- Inhibits growth of fungus
- Active against acne bacteria
- Used in treatment for vaginitis

# Terpineol

Smell/Taste: Diesel, Earthy, Floral, Herbal

Therapeutic Benefits

* Stops or kills airborne microorganisms from growing and causing disease
* Pain relief
* Reduces swelling/inflammation
* Destructive to bacteria
* Inhibits growth of fungus
* Blocks the sensation of pain to your brain, providing you pain relief
* Free radical scavenging activity
* Stops abnormal cell growth
* Inhibits growth of viruses
* Cell regenerative for skin, scar healing
* Counteracts gastric mucosal damage
* Lowers blood pressure
* Protects nerve cells against damage, degeneration or impairment function
* Calming

# Terpinolene

Smell/Taste: Diesel, Floral, Herbal

Therapeutic Benefits

  * Destructive to bacteria
  * Inhibits growth of fungus (Candida)
  * Free radical scavenging activity
  * Relieves spasms from voluntary or involuntary muscles
  * Inhibits growth of viruses
  * Calming

# Valencene

Smell/Taste: Earthy, Fruity, Herbal

Therapeutic Benefits

  * Skin Protectant

# CANNABIS WITH PRESCRIPTIONS

If you are currently on prescription medications, undergoing chemotherapy or radiation, and you are not under the care of a cannabis doctor, you should consult with a medical cannabis expert while taking these at the same time.

Chemo and radiation are dosed very specifically for you, your weight, the type of cancer you are being treated for, the severity of cancer and cannabis can affect your treatment. You must work with a specialist in this area to make sure you aren't interfering with your chemo and radiation or prescription drug dose.

Cannabis contains active compounds that work on receptors throughout your body. When you are taking prescription medications, they also attach to receptors. We want to make sure compounds in your cannabis products are not attaching to the same receptors as your prescriptions. If they are, this will affect the efficacy of your prescription making it more or less potent.

If you are on any prescription medications or have medical questions, and you are not working with a cannabis doctor, you can call the first cannabis nurse hotline Leaf411.

Website: www.leaf411.org

Phone: 1-844-LEAF411 (844-532-3411)

# CANNABIS WITH ALCOHOL

It is NOT recommended to be drinking alcohol of any percentage along with taking cannabis in any form.

Cannabis and alcohol do not mix well. When you have THC and alcohol working together, as my cannabis instructor Colleen Quinn would say, "it's like lighting a fire with gasoline. Your brain cannot handle it." It's not beneficial in any way. When they work together, they enhance the effects of THC by allowing THC to enter the brain more easily, and can possibly make you sick. Chose one or the other. If you are dealing with a health condition, I would choose cannabis out of the two options. Alcohol will not cure or improve your medical condition.

# CANNABIS AND PREGNANCY

Health experts agree that whether you are trying to get pregnant, pregnant or nursing, it's a good idea to discontinue use of CBD, Hemp and Cannabis to protect the health of the baby and the mother. There just isn't enough research to know the long term effects. I would even refrain from smoking hemp or cannabis around babies to 18 years old due to this being the critical years of brain development. You don't have to live in their body. Don't do something that could potentially affect them in the future.

# SUMMARY

I hope you have learned a lot and feel empowered with a purpose for your next visit to the dispensary. My goal with this quick guide to take to the dispensary was to get you more clear on your purpose and to feel comfortable when visiting the dispensary. The budtender will thank you if you are prepared to answer some questions on how they can better assist you on your healing journey.

Remember, it is YOUR body, and you get to heal in the way YOU want to. There are many options with cannabis and hemp and how you can use these plant products. Just know that there are products and routes that will be more effective if you take them properly, and in the properly spaced amount of time to keep that dose of cannabis in the therapeutic window of efficacy. Formulation also plays a big part in the efficacy of a product.

Let's get the most benefits from our plant medicine by following the instructions on how to take it. I need to close with one more real-life analogy. If you went to the doctor and you had pneumonia and they prescribed a bottle of antibiotics, and you were instructed to take 1 pill three times a day for 10 days, are you going to take 1 pill from the bottle, one time in the full ten days and think you will be cured? No, you will not.

There is a reason you take multiple pills for multiple days. You need to keep that antibiotic in the therapeutic window in your bloodstream so the antibiotics can work inside of you to do their job and kill off the pathogens.

Only taking one pill once, will not do the job. There is a reason behind dosing. To be effective it needs time inside your body to work and do its job. Listen to your body and take notes so you know what is working and what isn't so you can make adjustments.

And remember MORE is not always BETTER! START LOW and GO SLOW!


HAPPY HEALING!


*Jessica Faleide*
x♥x♥

# ABOUT THE AUTHOR

Jessica Faleide is the CEO/Founder of Organic Way of Life®, LLC, Cannabis With Class® and Hope for Healing™, LLC. She is a Clinical Aromatherapist, hemp and cannabis formulator, an Independent BEMER Distributor, Paramedical Aesthetician, author, and an aunt.

Jessica has always had a passion to help others heal externally and internally. She loves to read and share knowledge she has learned throughout the years and through her own health and healing journey. She has always wanted to inspire others to be their own health advocate and to be able to enjoy a long, fulfilling life without limitations.

She resides in North Dakota where she enjoys reading, waterskiing, wakeboarding, snowboarding, cross country skiing, swimming, kayaking, jet skiing, working in her yard, feeding the deer, working with dogs and horses, taking pictures of nature, and star gazing.

For more information, email jessica@cannabiswithclass.com
www.CannabisWithClass.com

Book information and downloadable guide at:
www.TakeMeToTheDispensary.com

YouTube Channel: Cannabis With Class

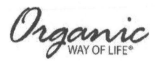

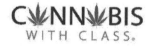

# *URGENT PLEA!*

## Thank You For Reading My Book!

I really appreciate all of your feedback and I love hearing what you have to say.

I need your input to make the next version of this book and my future books better.

Please take two minutes now to leave a helpful review on Amazon letting me know what you thought of the book.

https://amazon.com/review/create-review?&asin=B0BW2SDGRL

## Thank you very much!
Jessica Faleide

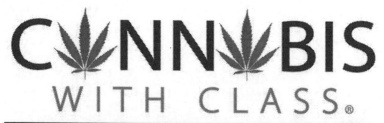

Your Official Cannabis With Class Apparel and Merchandise by Organic Way Of Life® ,LLC

**Featured Products**

# www.CannabisWithClass.com

Made in the USA
Columbia, SC
17 June 2023

17889490R00048